Ketogenic Diet

Table Of Contents

Introduction

This book contains proven steps and strategies on how to effectively prepare delicious, low-carb, and high-fat meals that will help the body transition into a lighter and leaner physique. It is expected that following a ketogenic-friendly meal plan, together with its nutritious recipes, will have a positive impact on one's longevity and quality of life.

The ketogenic diet's objective is to promote fat loss and weight management by following a healthy food ratio of high fat, moderate protein and very few carbs in our daily meals. This unique balance of carbs, protein and fat will subsequently trigger nutritional ketosis, a natural process that breaks down fat cells and turns it into energy.

In this book, the connection behind ketosis and weight loss will be explained in order to have greater appreciation for the ketogenic diet. You will likewise be able to see how a keto-adopted lifestyle affects blood sugar levels and prevents the onset of medical conditions that threaten one's health.

Moreover, the 70 recipes in this book that will help jumpstart a ketogenic lifestyle are categorized into 5 meals: breakfast, lunch, dinner, snack and dessert. Each recipe is easy to follow and uses natural yet low-carbohydrate ingredients that will satisfy your taste buds without adding extra inches on the waistline.

Thanks again for downloading this book, I hope you enjoy it!

Ketogenic Diet In A Nutshell

Every diet or eating lifestyle has its pro and cons alongside challenges that make first timers find it harder to adopt. Before we get to see what mistakes or pitfalls come with Ketogenic diet, let's first understand what the diet entails. In a nutshell, the ketogenic diet emphasizes on increasing your intake of fat and protein while reducing your intake of carbohydrates. The ketogenic diet is meant to restrict carbohydrate intake in order to control your blood sugar levels. Since our body's main source of energy is glucose, if your body is low in glucose, the body is forced to find other sources of energy to sustain the body's metabolism processes. Once under the "starvation" mode, your body is said to undergo ketosis. Simply put ketosis is a process in which the liver begins to synthesize ketone bodies and fatty acids as alternative sources of fuel. The stored fats are thereby broken down in the liver into fatty acids and other products that we now call ketone bodies. The ketone bodies are then oxidized as the main energy source to provide fuel for your body in place of carbohydrates.

The ketogenic diet was initially designed to help people suffering from epilepsy but with the availability of epileptic drugs, the diet is not as effective for those suffering from epilepsy. However, there has been a lot of success with the diet being effective in helping people lose weight. For you to lose weight with the Keto diet plan, you need to restrict your carb intake to less than 50g in a day. You should then meet your daily calorie requirement from food sources that offer high amounts of fats and lean protein to sustain metabolic processes. With that understanding of the ketogenic diet, let us now look at how you can lose weight with the ketogenic diet.

How The Ketogenic Diet works

The Ketogenic diet works by triggering a state of ketosis once your blood glucose levels are low. Ketosis is a body state in which you're at a high fat burning rate. Actually, the human brain normally runs on ketone bodies, the energy molecules found in the blood, which are processed from fat by the liver for fuel. A lower intake of carbohydrates can help trigger production of ketones bodies, and can also maintain lower levels of insulin secretion. It's important to sustain a lower insulin levels as it facilitates large amounts of ketones in the blood.

Even though low-carb intake is what is most important while on a ketogenic diet, you may at various occasions fail to achieve the maximum ketones in the blood mainly due to poor intake of proteins. And when I talk of poor protein intake it simply implies that you consume excess amounts of proteins say from fish, lean meat or seeds and nuts. The downside is that the excess protein is converted into glucose and can raise your insulin level at the expense of inhibiting ketosis. To avoid interfering with "optimal ketosis", just ensure that you eat more fat instead, as fat can induce satiety and fight cravings.

If your goal is to lose weight, you might be scared of eating a high fat diet but research has shown that healthy fatty foods like wild caught salmon, walnuts, and olive oil can actually facilitate weight loss.

Let us look at why you should adopt a ketogenic diet if you want to lose weight.

Advantages of Ketogenic Diet

Being in a state of ketosis has many benefits. If you suffer from diabetes or are pre-diabetic, obese or at the risk of developing heart disease adapting the Ketogenic diet can really help. Below are some of the benefits you get when on a low carb diet

Weight loss

Research has proven that dieters can actually lose weight while following a ketogenic diet. Actually, there have been reported cases where people have lost up to 160 pounds by switching to a ketogenic diet. A ketogenic diet serves to lower carbohydrate intake which forces your body to burn fat to produce energy. Due to the inefficiency of fat as a fuel, a lot of it has to be burned to release a relatively small amount of energy. Thus, ketosis can be very helpful in shedding that extra weight even if you are obese.

Lowers blood sugar levels

When we eat a high carb diet, the carbohydrates are broken down to glucose in the digestive tract where it is absorbed into the bloodstream. When it enters the bloodstream, it causes a spike in blood sugar and thus will force the body to produce more insulin to regulate the sugar levels. However, if you suffer from insulin resistance, your body is unable to regulate blood sugar levels and this might lead to type II diabetes. The ketogenic diet addresses this situation by lowering the amount of available glucose in the blood thus reducing the need for insulin.

Ketosis makes the body to utilize body fat for fuel

If you are on a high carbohydrate diet, the body breaks it down into glucose. The body will prefer to oxidize glucose rather than body fat since it uses less oxygen. On the other hand, ketosis makes the body efficient in burning your body fat instead so you can shed weight a lot faster. In addition, ketone bodies are very inefficient fuel and thus have very little calories relative to their mass. Therefore, if the body is in ketosis, it will burn a lot of fat in order to get adequate energy for a particular activity.

Ensures no excess fat is stored

Let's say your body has no use for excess ketones that are processed from fats, here it will simply excrete them out as urine. This is in contrast to a high carb diet where excess glucose is converted into fat and unfortunately stored "for later use". Therefore, a low carb diet does not only make it easier to lose body fat but also maintain body shape as no fat deposits are made.

Ketosis controls insulin levels

No doubt, a ketogenic diet helps lower your insulin levels to facilitate metabolism of fat into energy. Insulin has the ability to prevent the conversion of fat to energy; a process called lipolysis and a high carb diet increases the level of insulin and inhibits lipolysis. Thus, the lowered insulin levels will increase lipolysis hence more fat will be burned. In addition, the lowered insulin levels allows for the release of other beneficial hormones such as the growth hormone.

Helps burn abnormal fats

In a Ketogenic diet, majority of the fat that is burned is from the abdominal cavity what is referred to as visceral fat. As opposed to subcutaneous fat deposited under the skin, visceral fat can drive inflammation, insulin resistance and cause metabolic dysfunction. A low carb diet can help burn the visceral fat and thus can quickly get rid of that tummy fat.

While going on a ketogenic diet has many benefits, there are also downfalls to it. Let us look at some of the challenges you are likely to face while on ketosis.

Disadvantages of Ketosis

Ketosis may pose a few problems before you get used to the diet. However, you don't have to worry as most of these drawbacks are only temporary and can be corrected with time. For instance, you have to undergo a transition stage, as your body adjusts to using ketone bodies as a source of energy. Therefore, before then you may experience a number of side effects including fatigue, headaches, and nausea. Other drawbacks of the diet include:

Deficiency of micronutrients

Since foods rich in carbohydrates are restricted, you can have a deficiency of micronutrients that accompany these foods. Obviously this may lead to deficiency related conditions or diseases. However, this shouldn't worry you much as you can alternatively take vitamin and mineral supplements. Also remember to take a lot of fiber to aid in digestion, thus eat a lot of veggies.

Higher levels of cholesterol

Since the ketogenic diet requires increased intake of fats, it can cause the blood lipids to increase. This means instead of reducing cholesterol in the blood stream, the high intake of fats can cause the reverse effect of

increasing cholesterol levels. The good news is that unsaturated fatty foods like fish, nuts, seeds and beef can boost production
of the good HDL cholesterol.

Too high level of ketone bodies

There's a process referred to as Ketoacidosis in which the amount of ketone bodies multiplies and gets out of control. Such an outcome can then lead to acidosis, an effect which lowers the bloods pH, a condition that can be fatal if not treated. However, this is unlikely to affect non-diabetic people as their bodies keep blood sugar low and allow only enough ketones to be produced at any one time.

Hope by now you know how you stand to benefit by adopting the ketogenic diet and what to watch out for. In the following chapter, we are going to look at common pitfalls further and how to avoid them or recover from them.

Ketogenic Diet Pitfalls and How To Avoid Them

No doubt adopting a low-carb diet can be quite a challenge as a beginner especially if you are of the view that fat is a disaster to health and weight loss. That said; research has proven that reducing your carb intake and rather focusing on high fat and protein diet is the most efficient way to build muscle and lose weight. These two food groups have been studied to help dieters boost health and lower risks of diseases like diabetes, cancer, and cardiovascular problems.

That notwithstanding, a low-carb Ketogenic diet if implemented in a wrong manner can cause chronic inflammation, trigger hormonal imbalances and hinder weight loss. A common problem is the fact that many dieters don't differentiate between simple carbs from the complex carbs as well as how much carbohydrates they need to take to achieve ketosis as well as how their protein intake out to be. Imbalances in consumption of food groups can be addressed with prior knowledge on common pitfalls and how to avoid them. Let's see low-carb diet mistakes you should be aware of in advance:

Higher intake of carbs

By now you already know that you need to adopt a low-carb and high protein diet for weight loss but exactly what does low-carb translate to? Let's say your carb intake per day as an average American man sums up to 300 grams, reducing intake to 150 gram could be termed low-carb, right? You will be surprised that you need to go lower than that to around 20 percent of your carb calories intake! Research from American Journal of Clinical Nutrition has shown that for ketosis to take place uninterrupted, you need to maintain a carb intake of 50 grams daily.

If you live a sedentary lifestyle, 50grams intake of carbs may trigger sufficient production of ketone bodies and will cease to rely on glucose but stored fats for metabolism. The quick fix for a higher carb intake is to maintain a 50 gram intake of carbs by ensuring that you mainly consume dark-leafy green veggies. Remember that carbs don't only come from grains and processed foods but also from fruits and veggies. You need to check the carb content from fresh veggies before eating them, preferably celery, mushrooms, green beans, broccoli and lettuce. Don't be scared of eating salads often and ensure that you choose low-carb fruits and veggies. Since fruits could be rich in carbs, try selected fruits such as berries and practically avoid all grains, whether whole or processed.

Excess consumption of proteins

It's a fact that a higher intake of proteins can help boost satiety, lower cravings and actually help you get leaner as you lose weight. That said; excess intake of proteins than what your body actually requires can trigger gluconeogenesis, or the conversion of amino acids into glucose. Once this happens, the body's capability to burn fat is reduced as metabolism switches on glucose for fuel. A higher intake of 230 to 250 grams of proteins daily can hinder the body from excreting the toxic byproducts of protein metabolism such as ammonia. Furthermore, once the proteins aren't fully processed and get into the intestines, the undigested proteins undergo fermentation through the gut bacteria and yield inflammatory products. In extreme cases, protein only diet can cause loss of calcium and damage your kidneys.

So exactly how much proteins do your require? For those of you who workout, a 1.5-2.0 grams per each kilo of body weight can match well with a low-carb diet. Try to maintain protein intake to below 1.5 g/kg and ensure that the protein comes from animals and sea foods like fatty wild-caught salmon or kelp. You may also need to find out ketone concentration through a urine test even though the results might not reflect actual levels in the blood. The best way to check this out is through ketone blood test although it can be quite expensive.

Eating lesser calories from fat

The key concept of a ketogenic diet is to trigger your metabolism to burn fats rather than glucose in a bid to stop storage of fat in tissues. A lower fat intake can yield extremely low calorie intake, or cause elevated cortisol or reduced thyroid hormone functionality. What happens is when fat intake is lower than required, the production of energy is slowed down and you're unable to sustain a low-carb diet. The best way to make Ketogenic diet work is to ensure 50 percent of calories you eat come from fatty foods and oils.

The key to eating a high fat diet is to include fats at each meal, by choosing to consume fats from red-palm oil, olive oil, organic meats, fatty fish, avocados, nuts and olives. For breakfast, try the "fat coffee" trick by adding some oil, butter or heavy cream to your drink. For instance, you can add tablespoon of coconut oil and a tablespoon of butter to your morning or afternoon coffee. Blend to achieve the best consistency. The higher the fat intake, the lesser proteins and carbs you consume; which drops down insulin levels and gets you into optimal ketosis.

Also get fats by consuming fatty cuts of meat, cooked in butter if preferred, to facilitate conversion of fats and ketones for energy. Instead of just eating boneless and skinless chicken breast, try applying sufficient amounts of butter under the chicken leg skin and thigh before you cook. Use your fingers to wolf them as the butter drips your arms. Don't trim fats from your steaks but instead eat them the fatty side in. An easy way to get fats is eating bacon, and then eat it wobbly with its fat content intact.

Eating inadequate vegetables & fruit

Now that you know that even fruits and veggies have carbs, you might be tempted to eliminate all plant-based foods to maintain a 50 grams intake of carbs. However, be informed that veggies are nutrient-packed and plays a huge role in preventing diseases and curbing inflammatory reactions. Taking more veggies helps you boost your nutrients intake and reduces calories intake. You need to obtain around 5 servings daily of veggies either as a snack, main meal or a side dish. In addition to fruits and vegetables being high in nutrients, they are also high in fiber that promotes satiety and makes you eat less, thus you need them for fiber if you eliminate grains.

Ensure that you consume about 2-3 cups of carb veggies at each meal from low-glycemic carbs like green veggies, peppers, turnips, green beans, mushrooms, asparagus, egg plant, avocados, garlic and tomatoes. For fruits, ensure you limit their intake to fruits like berries to ensure you still get the important fiber and phytonutrients. A creative way to snack on fruits and veggies is to make your own salads. Also, consider healthy ingredients such as fresh herbs, balsamic vinegar, fresh lemon juice, Dijon mustard and extra-virgin olive oil for your dressing. Try this simple Soy-Ginger Dressing recipe: Whisk together 2 tablespoons of low-sodium soy sauce, minced garlic clove, 1½ teaspoon grated ginger and 2 tablespoons red wine vinegar. Then whisk the mixture into a ¼ cup of canola oil. The recommended serving size is 2 tablespoons per serving, with lesser amounts for creamier options. Try other ingredients like clove of garlic, roughly chopped scallions, mayonnaise, a medium avocado, fresh lemon juice, chopped fresh tarragon, chopped fresh parsley and chopped fresh basil. These can be blended to smoothness and then seasoned with freshly ground pepper and sea salt to taste.

Low intake of indigestible fiber

Research has shown that eating more animal proteins may cause you to eat less fiber particularly from fruits and veggies. It is important to note that dietary fiber doesn't raise your blood sugar level as it slows down glucose absorption into the blood. Fiber also makes you feel fuller for longer and fights cravings. A rule of the thumb is to consume 2-7 grams of fiber daily. Therefore, increase your fiber intake by 2-4 grams daily from consumption of veggies and fruits. Get soluble fiber from foods such as grapes, kiwi, pomegranates, blackberries, raspberries, tart cherries and blueberries. Low glycemic and fiber-rich veggies that should form your best choice include artichokes, asparagus, summer squash and broccoli.

You can also obtain best sources of fiber from fresh fruits, their seeds and pulp; though juicing fruits reduces their nutritional value. Try fiber-rich and low-glycemic fruits among them bananas, oranges, pears, peaches, water melon, grape fruit, green apples and berries. Lack of indigestible fiber from your diet can trigger inflammation from gut bacteria and cause chronic diseases, and not only fruits and veggies that support gut health but also probiotics like kefir, yoghurt, kim chi and sauerkraut. For instance you can choose to eat raw unmodified potato starch in that it triggers the synthesis of anti-inflammatory gut bacteria.

Going overboard with healthy fats

This applies to saturated fatty foods like coconut oil and butter alongside omega 3 fatty acids that are recommended in Ketogenic diet. Fats can strengthen your immune system and offer vitamins such as A, D and K in easily assimilated form. Though saturated fats are healthy if monitored, their excess consumption can lead to buildup of cholesterol that causes heart disease or even stroke. Research shows that high intake of saturated fats can raise LDL blood lipids that trigger cardiovascular inflammation. Regulate intake of such fats and oil to 1-2 tablespoons daily
can avoid buildup of plagues in arteries.

Other beneficial omega 3 fatty acids from foods like fish oil that is considered heart healthy ought to be monitored as excess consumption might lead to dysfunctional immune responses. A poor immunity can expose you to diseases, whereas consumption of oxidized omega-3 fats can damage your DNA. The oxidation in fish oil happens with poor quality fish oil since the omega-3 fatty acids are comprised of weak carbon double bonds. Ensure that you eat fatty fish 2-3 times a week, take few tablespoons of stabilized fish oil and eat food fortified or enriched with omega 3. Also lower intake of vegetable and oil based oils to control intake of omega 6 fats, say to a maximum of 10 grams a day.

Failure to monitor blood sugar

While it is true that while you are on a low-carb Ketogenic diet, your insulin levels and sugar tolerance should improve especially if suffering from diabetes, studies show that low-carb diets can make metabolic hormones like insulin and leptin to get out of balance. A chronic carb starvation or absence of insulin release can hinder leptin release, this hormone being the one that indicates satiety. Ever heard of carb cycling? It's advisable to eat carbs say every 5-7 days in order to maintain the cells sensitive to insulin and for the brain to be responsive to leptin hormone.

A problem can arise in case you consume a cheat meal say high carb or high-fat snack that can trigger release of excess glucose in the blood. That excess glucose can attach to protein molecules in what is referred to as glycation and lead to oxidative stress, which can eventually leads to different diseases. LDL cholesterol has a higher likelihood of being glycated and can lead to buildup of plague in the arteries or atherosclerosis. Even if you are on a low-carb diet, ensure that you regularly test your blood glucose levels. The results should help you determine your window to inflammation in your body; so try to maintain it to below 84 mg/dl.

A good way to avoid elevation of blood glucose in Ketogenic diet is to avoid high-carb cheat meals from refined foods. Instead of cheat meals or occasional high carb snacks, consider carb cycling that feature those whole unprocessed or complex carbs like fruits, squash, sweet potatoes and whole grains. It's also recommendable to have your hemoglobin A1C level determined in order to realize how your body handled glucose for the last 3 previous months. The test illustrates whether hemoglobin has been damaged by glycated glucose or not, so ensure that your results are below 5.5 percent.

Fasting while on low-carb diet

In an attempt to lose weight faster, you may want to combine a low carb diet and fasting for maximum results. While some people have experienced positive results with this combination, it may not be the best. When on a low carb diet, your sugar levels are low and your body turns to burning fat for energy. Even as you keep your sugar levels low by reducing your carbohydrate intake, it is important to avoid hypoglycemia. If you get to this point, your body will signal the adrenal glands to release cortisol and adrenaline. Cortisol, the stress hormone responsible for the "flight and fight" response will then signal the liver to convert any carbohydrates into glucose, which is then released to the blood stream. This is because your body thinks that you are in duress and you need all the glucose you can get to function. With consistently high glucose levels, your cells then crave for glucose and this can make the brain to trigger production of hormones for hunger. This will then leads to overeating, which is counterproductive.

Not getting enough essential minerals

Being on a low-carb diet and the state of ketosis can cause frequent urination, which go along with nutrients such as potassium, magnesium, and sodium. For instance electrolytes such as potassium and sodium are normally excreted along with ketones and a large amount of water as well. Lack of essential electrolytes can lead to low blood pressure, mineral imbalances and sluggishness. The symptoms of loss of electrolytes may be interpreted as low blood sugar and can cause you to give up on your low-carb diet.

The rule of the thumb during ketosis is to consume about 5000mg sodium daily, 300mg of magnesium and 100grams of potassium. A healthy diet can help you compensate for mineral requirements but in some cases, there's no need to take mineral supplements. On the other hand, supplementing with magnesium can lead to more complications for those people with kidney problems. Remember that magnesium is a co-factor in more than 300
enzymes in your body, and helps regulate a number of biochemical functions in your body. Magnesium is also required by the body to synthesize DNA and monitor heartbeat rate.

To increase the level of magnesium in the body, try using a cup of soymilk, ½ cup of boiled spinach, a medium banana, ½ cup of black beans and an ounce of cashew-nuts or almonds, roasted. And to get required potassium, ensure that you consume green veggies and also cook your meats together with broths. For sodium, you only need 2.5 to 3.5 grams of sodium so don't eat packaged or processed foods as these could be overloaded with sodium.

Not staying hydrated

A basic fact is that carbs attract water and facilitate the body to remain hydrated, and thus a low-carb diet can cause dehydration and strain the kidneys. Water also helps flush out toxins from the kidney and facilitate weight loss as toxins as usually stored as fat leading to weight gain. Many dieters on low-carb diet are afraid of water retention and thus regulate water intake in a bid to see immediate results on the scale. Though instant weight loss can impress you to stick to low-carb diet, the body quickly adjusts and instead adopts other ways of water retention. Did you know that dehydration also triggers cravings? It can also interrupt beta-oxidation process that deals with metabolism of fats as energy sources. In case you regularly take a few cups of coffee daily, ensure you also consume a few glasses say 6-8 of pure and plain water as well. And for beer lovers, it's good that you moderate your intake or avoid alcohol altogether, even whisky or red wine!

Having too many cheat days

Let's face it, it can be hard to fully forsake your sweet tooth, and thus occasionally you can choose to eat a few sugary snacks. However, eating a high carb snack hinders ketosis and slows down weight loss. Furthermore, carbs (especially simple carbs) cause cravings for more carbs as it alters your brain's hunger detention mechanism! The key is to try harder not to cheat and also avoiding those packaged low-carb foods as they are likely to be loaded with sugar alcohol. This substance is an addictive that can elevate sugar level in your metabolism due to its high glycemic index. Using such packed "healthy" products can cause hormonal imbalance and hinder effective weight loss.

You can adopt various creative ways to snack and enjoy what you eat without going overboard, if only you have prepared snacks regularly. For instance, the protein-rich nuts, hard cheese slices, or hard-boiled eggs can come in handy. Normally, we would want to have a cheat meal especially when we don't have much to eat around the house. Therefore, avoid these instances by ensuring that there is always a healthy meal. Did you know that leftovers could help simplify your life especially if served as lunch or snack? Therefore, always have some leftovers for the following day to ensure that you always have healthy foods at hand and this will avoid instances of wanting a cheat meal.

Also ensure that you eat at least 2 low-carb snacks per day especially after breakfast, after lunch and dinner, to help remain fuller. For additional snack options, try taking nuts, tuna, smoked salmon, hard-boiled eggs, leftover diced pork chops, leftover pulled chicken or taco meat. Ensure to use fats when dressing salads; and use enzyme-rich mayonnaise or sour cream combined with healthy oils for a creamy taste. Try Asian snacks among them dried anchovies and kelp chips prepared in coconut or palm oil. You can also fry your own snacks, by simply frying cheese in bacon grease or coconut oil. Also fry veggies such as peppers and onions in lard or coconut oil until crisp. Remember to add in some herbs and spices, like garlic and black pepper.

Not exercising regularly

Regardless of how a low-carb diet can facilitate detox and weight loss, you need to adopt a physically fit lifestyle as well. Research shows that altering diet only works for few dieters, and soon the body will adapt to the diet and you reach a weight loss plateau!

Exercising can help trigger synthesis of proteins and can inhibit your body from utilizing the muscle mass for fat loss. Workouts such as aerobic exercising can help the body metabolize fats for energy especially if you're already obese or living a sedentary lifestyle. Interval exercises can also help you burn fats, reduce bad cholesterol, control blood sugar and strengthen the heart and lungs. Even if you are busy most of the day, try to have at least 20 minutes of interval training per day.

Ways to exercise can involve constant movement like walking let's say amid a normal chat to a friend. Here you can do 5 minutes warm up before doing interval training; and rest for 5 minutes to allow cooling down. Alternatively, you can choose to walk at a brisk pace, where you can still manage a conversation amid breathing faster. For better results, try to move or walk at a faster pace. In case it's a weekend, try more challenging workouts like biking, swimming or other top speed activity. Ensure that once your fitness improves that you increase your speed and resistance to match your new level.

Eating excessive nuts

Nuts are good snack options and can help you avoid eating processed foods that wreck havoc on insulin production and fat metabolism. However, failure to monitor the amounts of nuts you snack on can be a problem since not all nuts are the same. For instance based on calorie levels, chestnuts, pistachios and cashew nuts are the worst in terms of their calorie content. These nuts could be full of heart-healthy fats but eating half a bag in a day can leads to giving your body excess calories than what it actually needs. You will be surprised to learn that, just 100 grams of cashew nuts has a whooping 550 calories! In case you love nuts and can't get over it, try to store them away from you; and then only carry a few with you to help track intake.

Chapter 1:
Ketogenic Diet: Triggering Weight Loss One Less Carb at a Time

The more fat you have on your body,

the longer you can survive.

If we had to rely on glucose, we'd die in a few days.

Dr. Peter Attia

Co-founder of Nutrition Science Initiative;

Ketogenic diet advocate

The ketogenic diet is a low-carbohydrate, high-fat and moderate-protein diet that aims to help people shed unwanted pounds, thus resulting to a leaner and slimmer physique. This diet focuses on reducing carbs in order to prevent the rise of blood sugar, insulin, and triglyceride levels which are the major culprits of persistent weight gain and visceral fat production.

Under the ketogenic diet, the following is a nutritional ratio that can effectively trigger fat loss and promote long-term weight management:

Fat – 150 grams per day, or 73% of total daily consumption

Protein – 90 grams per day, or 20% total daily consumption

Carbohydrates – 30 grams per day, or 7% total daily consumption

This implies that adopting a ketogenic lifestyle requires us to drastically reduce our carbohydrate intake and incorporate more healthy fats into our meals in order for the body to undergo nutritional ketosis, a process wherein the body derives energy from fat cells instead of sugar.

The Science behind Ketosis and Weight Loss

Once the body starts to consume fewer carbohydrates from food such as rice, bread or potatoes, lesser glucose is released into the bloodstream. High levels or blood sugar and insulin, the body's conventional sources of fuel, are dramatically reduced. At this stage, transitioning to a ketogenic diet may initially cause weakness and intense cravings as energy sources within the body change.

However, the absence of carbs and sugars subsequently allows nutritional ketosis to take over the energy production process within the body. The moment that stored bodily fat cells are broken into energy, the body becomes leaner, lighter and more effective at performing weight loss activities such as cardio exercises and weight training

Moreover, once the body becomes ketogenic-adapted, you will find that cravings for carbohydrates will reduce and the body will be looking forward to eating cleaner and healthier food such as vegetables, fruits, meat and oils. As a result, symptoms of lifestyle diseases such as diabetes, heart disease, chronic pain and obesity will become easier to manage or eliminate.

Based on the natural effects of ketosis, the ketogenic diet is a more effective weight loss tool than other low-carb or calorie-restrictive diets: it does not only trigger fat loss and high energy levels but it also prevents the onset of medical conditions that threaten people's health and longevity. Through proper nutrition and smarter food choices, the ketogenic diet will help the body achieve a total transformation which will significantly improve the quality of life.

Foods to Eat For Effective Ketosis

People who are unfamiliar with the ketogenic diet tend to pre-judge this healthy meal plan as difficult to maintain mainly because organic foods are seemingly hard to find and a bit more expensive than the usual items seen at the grocery store.

On the contrary, a ketogenic meal plan consists of low-carb vegetables, eggs, dairy, fruits, meats, seafood and healthy oils that can be easily found in the outer lanes of the grocery or among the colorful, healthy crates of organic
food items at your local market. Natural spices and organic sweeteners can be used to add flare to ketogenic recipes, hence making these dishes more flavorful than your usual take-outs or microwaveable dinners.

Moreover, organic ingredients are reasonably-priced in comparison with high-carb meal options such as rice dinners, boxed pizza or fast food. Apart from saving you money, a keto lifestyle also promotes creativity in the kitchen by encouraging you to combine cheap but healthy ingredients in order to create a weight-friendly daily meal plan.

While organic food are at the top of the list, the ketogenic diet discourages the high consumption of natural carbs such as rice, high-carb vegetables, bread, grains, fruits and legumes as these tend to spike-up blood sugar levels. It is important to keep the carbohydrate ratio low so that you do not fall off the ketogenic wagon and gain even more weight.

The succeeding chapter contains a complete one-week meal plan that will serve as your initial guide in ketogenic meal preparation. Hopefully this will help you in your journey towards healthier living and long-term weight loss.

Chapter 2:
Comprehensive 7-Day Ketogenic Meal Plan for Beginners

Creating a weekly ketogenic meal plan may take a bit more time than the usual, but once you master the carbohydrate-fat-protein ratio then you will find that transitioning to a keto lifestyle is as simple as adopting a portion-controlled, organic way eating.

Here is a comprehensive 7-day ketogenic meal plan that will give you an idea on how to create a balanced set of nutritious dishes throughout the day.

Day 1

Breakfast – Parmesan, Ham and Basil Omelet

Lunch – Keto-Friendly Fried Chicken

Snack – Spicy Baked Zucchini Chips

Dinner – Coconut Fish Fingers with Garlic Mayo Dip

Dessert – Frozen Watermelon Creamsicles

Day 2

Breakfast – Spicy and Savory Breakfast Patties

Lunch – Fiery Egg Drop Soup

Snack – Baked Coconut Crisps

Dinner – Wheat-Free Pork and Veggie Sandwich

Dessert – Luscious Coconut Brownies

Day 3

Breakfast – High-Fiber Keto Oatmeal

Lunch – Low-Carb Tuna Avocado Meatballs

Snack – Garlicky Pork Chips

Dinner – Oven-Baked Rib-eye Steak

Dessert – Coconut Pudding with Fresh Berries

Day 4

Breakfast – Energizer Green Smoothie

Lunch – Spiced Pork Chops with Stir-Fried Veggies

Snack – Crispy Brussels Sprouts with Hot Mayo Sauce

Dinner – Low-Carb Vegetarian Pan Pizza

Dessert – Watermelon & Cucumber Sorbet

Day 5

Breakfast – Fully Loaded Breakfast Frittata

Lunch – Low-Carb Bacon Meatball Skewers

Snack – Light and Healthy Spinach Crackers

Dinner – Grilled Tilapia Fillet with Arugula Salad

Dessert – Almond Coconut Fat Bombs

Day 6

Breakfast – Crunchy Sunflower Seed Cereal

Lunch – Low-Carb Zucchini Carbonara

Snack – Cheesy Baked Sugar Snap Peas

Dinner – Quick and Easy Grilled Chicken Teriyaki

Dessert – Heavenly Chocolate Bacon Strips

Day 7

Breakfast – Sunny Tangerine Smoothie

Lunch – Summer Tomato, Cucumber and Shrimp Salad

Snack – Extra Spicy Devilled Eggs

Dinner – Slow-Braised Oxtail Stew

Dessert – Chocolate Peppermint Bark

The complete recipes of the dishes listed on this 7-day meal plan are found on the succeeding chapters. In addition, there are 35 more ketogenic recipes included in this book in order to give you more options and creativity for your meals.

Chapter 3:
Breakfast Recipes

Make yourself a low-carb breakfast such as scrambled eggs, lean meat burgers or fruit smoothies: this will provide you with intense energy throughout the day and supply your body with the right nutrients needed for that morning workout.

1. Parmesan, Ham and Basil Omelet

Ingredients:

4 large eggs

1½ tablespoons freshly-chopped basil leaves

¾ cup grated parmesan cheese

2 thin slices of cooked ham, minced

1 small avocado, pitted and sliced

2 tablespoons coconut oil

Pinch of sea salt

Directions:

Whisk together the eggs and parmesan cheese. Add in the basil, ham and sea salt. Mix well.

Heat the coconut oil in a pan over medium-high flame. Once the oil is hot, pour in the egg mixture and cook for 30 seconds. To prevent the egg from burning, use a spatula to push the sides of the egg towards the center.

Flip the omelet and cook the other side for 1 minute. Once the omelet is cooked, remove it from the heat and transfer it to a serving plate.

Top the omelet with avocado slices and serve.

This recipe yields 2 servings.

2. Sunny Tangerine Smoothie

Ingredients:

3 cups full-fat coconut milk

4 tablespoons shredded coconut

5 tangerines, peeled and deseeded

2 teaspoons tangerine zest

½cup fresh lime juice

½teaspoon vanilla

3 cups ice cubes

Directions:

Pour the coconut milk and lime juice in a blender and pulse. Add in the shredded coconut, tangerines, zest, vanilla and ice cubes and blend the smoothie for 10-15 seconds.

Pour the smoothie into glasses and serve immediately.

This recipe yields 4 servings.

3. Energizer Green Smoothie

Ingredients:

1 avocado, peeled, pitted and sliced

3 cups spinach leaves

1½ tablespoons roasted flaxseed

1½ cups almond milk

1 cup coconut milk

4 drops liquid stevia

3 ice cubes

Directions:

Place the avocado, spinach, flaxseed, almond milk, coconut milk, stevia and ice cubes in a blender and process until the desired consistency is met.

Pour the smoothie into glasses and serve immediately.

This recipe yields 2 servings.

4. Microwaveable Bacon and Egg Biscuit

Ingredients:

2 large eggs

4 tablespoon flaxseed meal

2 tablespoons coconut flour

2 teaspoons unsalted butter

1 teaspoon baking powder

Pinch of sea salt

3 bacon strips, cooked until golden brown

2 sunny-side up cooked eggs

Directions:

In a mixing bowl, blend together the flour, flaxseed, salt and baking powder. Add in the butter and slowly mix it into the flour mixture with a fork. The flour mixture should have a crumbly appearance.

Beat 2 large eggs in a separate bowl then slowly pour into the flour mixture. With a wooden spoon, mix the ingredients together until a smooth batter forms.

Divide the batter by pouring it into 2 greased 4-inch ramekins. Place the ramekins in a microwave and cook it on high for 1 minute. Once the biscuits are done, let it cool then remove it from the ramekins.

Slice each biscuit vertically in the middle. Place equal amounts of bacon and egg in between each biscuit then serve immediately.

This recipe yields 2 servings.

5. <u>Savory Green Waffles</u>

Ingredients:

1 bunch spinach, washed, drained and chopped

4 eggs

3 bacon strips, cooked and chopped

1 tablespoon full-fat coconut milk

Pinch of salt and black pepper
Directions:

Place the coconut milk and eggs in a bowl then whisk them together. Gradually fold in the chopped spinach and mix well. Season the egg mixture with salt and pepper.

Grease the waffle iron with cooking spray and turn on the heat. Pour the egg mixture into the heated pan and sprinkle chopped bacon on top. Close the waffle iron and let the dish cook for 3 minutes. Once the waffle is cooked, use a fork to remove it from the pan and transfer it to a serving plate.

This recipe yields 2 servings.

6. Early Riser's Muffin Sandwich

Ingredients:

4 large eggs

200 grams breakfast sausage

½ cup chicken stock

4 tablespoons melted unsalted butter

Pinch of sea salt and black pepper

Hot sauce

Directions:

To make the muffin loaves, pour 2 tablespoons of butter on a frying pan over medium flame. Once the butter begins to heat up, place 4 round biscuit cutters on the pan. Place an egg into each biscuit cutter then prick the yolks with a fork. Sprinkle each egg with salt and pepper.

Slowly pour the chicken stock into the pan, making sure that the liquid stays outside the biscuit cutters. Cover the pan, adjust the flame to low and cook the eggs for 3-4 minutes. Once the eggs are cooked, slowly remove them from the pan and let it cool.

To make the sausage patty, pour the remaining butter onto the pan and heat it up over medium flame. Create 2 thick and round patties with the breakfast sausage then place them on the pan. Cook each side for 3 minutes.

To assemble the sandwich, place 2 eggs on a plate. Place a sausage patty over each egg, squeeze some hot sauce over it then cover each patty with the remaining eggs.

This recipe yields 2 servings.

7. Crunchy Sunflower Seed Cereal

Ingredients:

1 ½ cups raw sunflower seeds

1 ½ tablespoons ground cinnamon

2 cups coconut shreds

1 teaspoon coconut oil

½teaspoon sea salt

2 medium eggs

½cup organic honey

2 cups full-fat coconut milk, chilled

Directions:

Prepare a parchment-lined baking sheet and preheat the oven to 350 °
F.

Grind the sunflower seeds and coconut shreds in a food processor.
Once both ingredients are fully chopped, add in the eggs, honey, salt,
cinnamon and coconut oil. Process the mixture for 1-2 minutes.

Using a spatula, place the mixture into the baking sheet and press
downwards and sideways for an even thickness. Place the cereal in the
oven and bake for 15 minutes.

Once the cereal is ready, remove it from the oven and let it cool for 20
minutes. Use a wooden spoon to lightly tap and break the cereal into
small bits.

Place the cereal into individual bowls and pour the chilled coconut
milk on top of it. Serve immediately.

This recipe makes 2 servings.

8. Keto-Friendly Pancakes and Bacon Strips

Ingredients:

10 bacon slices, cooked

1 cup almond flour

½cup coconut flour

5 large eggs

½ teaspoon baking soda ¼ cup coconut milk

¼ cup water

12 drops liquid stevia ¼ cup Erythritol

¼ cup egg white protein

½ cup melted unsalted butter Directions:

Whisk together the eggs, coconut milk, water and liquid stevia. Set this
aside.

In another bowl, mix together the almond flour, coconut flour, baking
soda, Erythritol and egg white protein.

Slowly pour the egg mixture into the dry ingredients. Mix the pancake
batter thoroughly.

Heat the butter in a pan over medium flame. Using a wooden spoon,
pour a strip of batter into the pan, making sure its shape mimics the
shape of the bacon strip. Place a strip of bacon in the middle of the

pancake and wait for the sides to bubble. Flip the pancake and continue cooking for a minute or two. Follow the same process for the remaining batter until you have 10 bacon pancakes. Serve warm.

This recipe yields 5 servings.

9. **Spicy and Savory Breakfast Patties**

Ingredients:

900 grams ground chicken meat

1 large egg, beaten

1 teaspoon garlic powder

2 teaspoon sea salt

1 teaspoon onion powder

½ teaspoon fresh thyme ¼ teaspoon chili flakes

1 teaspoon ground black pepper

1 teaspoon chopped parsley ¼ teaspoon nutmeg

¼ teaspoon paprika

2 teaspoons chopped dried sage

3 tablespoons olive oil

Directions:

Place the ground chicken and egg in a bowl and mix well. Gradually blend in the garlic powder, salt, onion powder, thyme, sage, nutmeg, paprika and chili flakes into the chicken mixture. Form the spiced mixture into 16 round patties then set aside.

Heat the olive oil in a pan over medium flame. Place the patties on the hot oil and cook for 3-5 minutes. Flip each patty over and cook the remaining side for 3 minutes. Place the breakfast patties on a plate and serve while hot.

This recipe yields 8 servings.

10. **Fruit and Greens Breakfast Bowl**

Ingredients:

2 cups kale leaves, stems discarded

2 scoops protein powder

4 tablespoons coconut cream

1 cup almond milk

2 tablespoons melted coconut oil

4 ice cubes

1 tablespoon shredded coconut

2 tablespoons ground almonds

2 teaspoons chia seeds

Slices of banana

Directions:

Place the kale leaves, whey protein, coconut cream, almond milk, coconut oil and ice cubes in a blender.

Process for 20 seconds then pour the contents in a bowl.

Sprinkle the ground almonds, shredded coconut and chia seeds on top of the cereal. Top with banana slices and serve.

This recipe yields 2 servings.

11.   **Herbed Bacon and Egg Cups**

Ingredients:

½tablespoon chopped fresh chives

½tablespoon chopped fresh parsley

12 bacon strips

8 eggs

½cup cottage cheese

½cup shredded cheddar cheese

2 jalapeno peppers, deseeded and minced

½ teaspoon garlic powder

Pinch of salt and ground black pepper
 Olive oil

Directions:

Lightly grease 12 muffin cups with olive oil and set aside. Preheat the oven to 350 ° F.

Place the bacon in a pan over medium flame and cook until light golden brown but not crispy. Cool the bacon for 2 minutes, then place a strip inside each muffin cup, circling the sides of the vessel. Set aside.

Whisk together the eggs, chives, parsley, cheeses, jalapeno peppers, garlic powder, salt and pepper in a mixing bowl. Pour the egg mixture into each bacon-lined cup, making sure that some space is left on the top so as to prevent the egg from overflowing.

Bake the egg cups for 25 minutes. Serve immediately.

This recipe yields 12 servings.

12.   High-Fiber Keto Oatmeal

Ingredients:

4 cups coconut milk

¾ cup flaxseeds

1 cup ground almonds

½cup finely-chopped cauliflower

½cup cottage cheese

¼ cup heavy cream

3 tablespoons unsalted butter, melted

1 teaspoon cinnamon powder

¼ teaspoon allspice ½ teaspoon vanilla ½ teaspoon nutmeg

10 drops liquid stevia

3 tablespoons Erythritol Directions:

Pour the coconut milk inside a saucepan and mix in the cauliflower. Heat the mixture over medium-high flame.

Once the mixture starts to boil, season it with cinnamon, allspice, vanilla and nutmeg. Mix well. Gradually add in the stevia, Erythritol and flaxseeds and mix until the oatmeal starts to thicken.

Pour the melted butter, cottage cheese and heavy cream into the oatmeal mixture and continue cooking for 5 minutes. Turn off the heat then spoon the oatmeal into individual bowls. Sprinkle chopped almonds on top of each bowl of oatmeal. Serve while hot.

This recipe yields 6 servings.

13.   Bacon and Eggs in a Basket

Ingredients:

7 medium eggs

7 bacon slices, chopped

1 cup finely-chopped tomatoes

2 cups grated sharp cheddar cheese

26

3 tablespoons olive oil
½ teaspoon salt

1 teaspoon paprika

½ teaspoon cayenne pepper Directions:

Preheat the oven to 400 ° F and line a baking sheet with parchment paper. Prepare an upside down muffin tin that will mold the cheese baskets.

To make the baskets, place 7 equal mounds of cheddar cheese on the baking sheet and sprinkle it with cayenne pepper and paprika. Bake the cheese mounds in the oven for 10 minutes.

Remove the cheese from the oven and slowly place them on top of the upside-down muffin pan, letting the sides fall slightly but not detach from the base. Let it cool and harden at room temperature.

While the cheese baskets are setting, heat the olive oil in a pan over medium-high flame. Fry each egg in a sunny-side up manner then set aside. Sprinkle some salt over each egg.

Once the eggs are done, cook the chopped bacon in the same pan until it becomes golden brown.

To assemble the dish, place 1 cheese basket on a plate. Place an egg over the basket followed by half a teaspoon of bacon. Top each basket with some chopped tomatoes and serve immediately.

This recipe yields 7 servings.

14.   **Fully-Loaded Breakfast Frittata**

Ingredients:

12 eggs

2 cups sharp cheddar cheese, grated

6 cups kale leaves, washed and drained

1 small onion, chopped

1 green bell pepper, deseeded and chopped

4 tablespoons coconut milk

4 tablespoons heavy cream

200 grams breakfast sausage

200 grams chorizo, casing discarded

1 teaspoon garlic powder

1 tablespoon olive oil

Pinch of sea salt

Directions:

Place the kale leaves, onions, bell peppers and olive oil in a pan and cook the vegetables on medium-high flame for 5 minutes. Remove the veggies from the heat and transfer it to a large mixing bowl.

In the same pan, cook together the sausage and chorizo until the meat becomes golden brown. Once the meat is cooked, transfer it into the bowl of cooked vegetables. Add in the cheddar cheese and mix the ingredients together. Set aside.

Whisk together the eggs, coconut milk and heavy cream. Season it with garlic powder and salt. Pour the egg mixture into the bowl of vegetables, cheese and meat. Blend the ingredients well.

Pour the frittata mixture into a lightly greased skillet and place it in the oven. Bake the frittata for 45 minutes inside a 350 ° F oven.

Let the frittata cool for 10 minutes then slice into squares. Serve warm.

This recipe yields 20 servings.

Chapter 4:
Lunch Recipes

B reak that mid-day hunger by eating a light, ketogenic lunch. Whether you have a veggie salad, soup or a plate of lean pork chops, a low-carb lunch will help keep the stomach full and maintain energy for mid-day activities such as lunch meetings or household chores.

1. Spiced Pork Chops with Stir-Fried Veggies

Ingredients:

3 large pork chops

2 teaspoons cumin

1 teaspoon coriander

1 teaspoon garlic powder

¼ cup flaxseed

Pinch of salt and ground black pepper

1 yellow bell pepper, deseeded and chopped

2 celery stalks, chopped

1 white onion, chopped

1 tablespoon butter

3 tablespoons olive oil

Directions:

In a bowl, mix together the cumin, coriander, flaxseed and garlic powder. Dip each pork chop into the spice mixture, making sure that all sides are evenly coated. Set aside.

Heat the olive oil in a pan over medium-high flame. Add the pork chops to the hot oil and cook for 3-5 minutes. Flip the pork chops over and cook the other side for 3 minutes. Remove the meat from the heat and let it cool for 5 minutes.

In another pan, heat the butter over medium flame. Add in the celery, bell peppers and onions and stir-fry the vegetables for 3 minutes. Turn off the heat.

Place the stir-fried vegetables on a plate. Arrange the pork chops on top of the vegetables. Serve immediately.

This recipe yields 3 servings.

2. Keto-Friendly Egg Salad

Ingredients:

3 pre-boiled eggs, cooled and peeled

3 lettuce leaves (Romaine or Iceberg)

1 teaspoon Dijon mustard

½teaspoon fresh lemon juice

1 ½ tablespoon mayonnaise

1 teaspoon olive oil

½teaspoon paprika

Pinch of salt and ground black pepper

Directions:

Place the eggs in a food processor and pulse until the eggs are roughly chopped. Gradually mix in the mayonnaise, mustard and lemon juice then blend for 10 seconds. Open the food processor then season the egg mixture with paprika, salt and pepper. Blend the salad for 5-10 seconds, depending on the preferred creaminess of the mixture.

Arrange the lettuce leaves on a serving plate. Spoon the egg salad onto the bed of lettuce then drizzle olive oil on top before serving.

This recipe yields 2 servings.

3. Fiery Egg Drop Soup

Ingredients:

4 eggs

3 cups homemade chicken broth

1 cup coconut milk

1 tablespoon butter

½ chicken bouillon

1 ½ teaspoons red chili flakes

Directions:

In a large saucepan over medium-high flame, boil together the chicken broth, bouillon and butter. Stir occasionally. Lower the flame once the stock starts to bubble.

One by one, crack the eggs into the steaming stock. Pour in the coconut milk then season it with red chili flakes. Stir the soup for 2 minutes then turn off the flame. Continue stirring for another 2 minutes or until the soup starts to thicken. Pour into bowls and serve while hot.

This recipe yields 4 servings.

4. Chunky Avocado and Tomato Salad

Ingredients:

2 large avocadoes, peeled and pitted

500 grams tomatoes

4 cups chopped lettuce

10 bacon slices, fried and chopped

¾ cup mayonnaise

Pinch of salt and black pepper

Directions:

Slice the avocadoes and tomatoes into ½ inch chunks and place them in a salad bowl. Mix in the lettuce and mayonnaise then toss the ingredients together. Season the salad with salt and pepper. Sprinkle the chopped bacon on top before serving.

This recipe yields 4 servings.

5. Summer Tomato, Cucumber and Shrimp Salad

Ingredients:

1 heirloom tomato, diced

450 grams cooked shrimp, diced

1 medium cucumber, peeled and diced
 1 tablespoon bottled capers

2 tablespoons mayonnaise

2 teaspoons Dijon mustard

½ cup lemon juice

Pinch of sea salt and black pepper

½teaspoon fresh dill

2 cups mixed greens Directions:

Arrange the mixed greens in a salad bowl and set aside.

In a separate bowl, toss together the tomatoes, cucumbers, shrimp, capers, mustard, mayonnaise and lemon juice. Season the tossed salad with salt and pepper.

Pour the salad into the bowl of mixed greens and sprinkle fresh dill on top. Chill the salad in the refrigerator for an hour then serve.

This recipe yields 3 servings.

6. Keto-Friendly Fried Chicken

Ingredients:

2 chicken breasts, sliced and opened up

2 large eggs, beaten

¾cup shredded parmesan cheese

1 cup ground pork rinds

2 tablespoons coconut oil

Pinch of salt and ground black pepper Directions:

Mix together the parmesan, pork rinds, salt and pepper in a bowl.

In a separate bowl, place the beaten eggs. Heat the coconut oil in a pan over medium-high flame.

Dip each chicken breast into the egg mixture then place it into the pork rind bowl to coat it. After that, dip the chicken into the egg mixture again and roll it into the rind mixture.

Place the coated chicken into the pan of hot oil and cook each side for 6-8 minutes. You may lower the heat once you have flipped the chicken over.

This recipe yields 2 servings.

7. Low-Carb Tuna Avocado Meatballs

Ingredients:

280 grams canned tuna fish, drained

1 medium avocado, peeled, pitted and diced

1 cup chopped celery

¼cup cottage cheese

¼cup mayonnaise

¼teaspoon onion powder

¼teaspoon paprika
 1/3 cup almond flour

1 cup olive oil

Pinch of salt and ground black pepper

Directions:

Transfer the tuna to a mixing bowl and season it with salt, onion powder, paprika and pepper. Mix well.

Add in the avocado, celery, cheese and mayonnaise. Slightly mash the ingredients together. Form 12 meatballs from the tuna avocado mixture then roll it in the almond flour. Set aside.

Heat the olive oil in a pan over medium-high flame. Once the oil is hot, fry the meatballs until the sides are golden brown. Let it cool for 5 minutes then serve.

This recipe yields 12 meatballs

8. Hot and Spicy Pork Taco Wraps

Ingredients:

10 iceberg or Boston lettuce leaves, washed and drained

400 grams lean ground pork

1 cup tomato salsa

½ teaspoon garlic powder ¼ teaspoon cumin

½ teaspoon onion powder

¼ teaspoon ground black pepper

1 tablespoon olive oil

Slices of avocado, bell peppers and red onions Directions:

Place the ground pork, garlic powder, cumin, onion powder and black pepper in a bowl. Using your hands, knead the spices into the meat.

Heat the olive oil in a skillet over medium flame. Place the spiced ground pork on the skillet and cook it until the meat becomes brown.

Once the meat is cooked, turn off the flame and drain the excess oil from the cooked pork. Pour the salsa over the pork and mix well.

To assemble the taco wraps, place a lettuce leaf on a plate, spoon the pork mixture on top of it then place some chopped avocadoes, peppers and onions. Fold or roll the lettuce leaf to secure the pork inside it. Serve immediately.

This recipe yields 2 servings.

9. Low-Carb Bacon Meatball Skewers

Ingredients:

5 bacon slices

450 grams ground pork

½teaspoon salt

½teaspoon ground black pepper

½teaspoon onion powder

½teaspoon garlic powder
½ teaspoon turmeric powder

½cup olive oil

Chunks of tomato, cucumber and pineapple

Directions:

Place the bacon and ground pork in a food processor and blend well. Season the meatball mixture with salt, pepper, onion powder, garlic powder and turmeric powder.

Form the mixture into 20 meatballs and place it on a parchment-lined baking sheet. Bake the meatballs in a 170 ° F oven for 12 minutes. Let the meatballs cool on a wire rack for 10 minutes.

To serve, place a chunk of tomato, cucumber, pineapple and meatball through a small skewer. Place the skewers on a serving plate and drizzle with olive oil.

This recipe yields 10 servings.

10. Zesty Chili Crab Cakes

Ingredients:

3 cups fresh crab meat

2 large eggs

2 tablespoon coconut flour

4 tablespoons minced green chilies

1 tablespoon minced garlic

1 teaspoon Dijon mustard

½ teaspoon mayonnaise

Pinch of sea salt and black pepper

3 tablespoons olive oil

Directions:

In a large bowl, mix together the crab meat, eggs, chilies, garlic, mustard and mayonnaise. Season the mixture with salt and pepper then gradually add the coconut flour to thicken its consistency. Mix well.

Form the mixture into 10 round patties and set aside.

Heat the olive oil in a large pan over medium-high flame. Place the crab cakes on the pan and cook each side for 3 minutes or until golden brown.

This recipe yields 10 servings.

11. Crunchy Greens and Pine Nuts Salad

Ingredients:

Directions:

1 cup arugula

1 cup spinach

3 iceberg lettuce leaves, torn

3 tablespoons toasted pine nuts

3 bacon slices, cooked

1 cup shredded parmesan cheese

2 tablespoons lemon juice
2 tablespoons olive oil

Pinch of salt and ground black pepper

Directions:

Wash and pat dry the arugula, spinach and lettuce leaves. Place them in a salad bowl.

Chop the bacon into small pieces then add these on top of the greens. Sprinkle the pine nuts and parmesan cheese on top of the salad. Set aside.

In a small bowl, whisk together the olive oil, lemon juice, salt and pepper. Pour the dressing into the salad bowl and toss the ingredients together. Place the salad in the refrigerator for 1 hour.

This recipe yields 3 servings.

12. Roasted Cauliflower and Pepper Chowder

Ingredients:

1 small head of cauliflower, cut into small florets

2 green bell peppers, halved and deseeded

3 green onions, minced

2 tablespoons olive oil

4 tablespoons butter

½teaspoon red pepper flakes

½cup coconut cream

3 cups homemade chicken broth

1 teaspoon garlic powder

1 teaspoon paprika

1 teaspoon chopped fresh thyme

Pinch of salt and ground black pepper

Directions:

Preheat the oven to 400 ° F and line 2 baking sheets with parchment paper.

Arrange the pepper halves on a baking sheet. Meanwhile, place the cauliflower florets on the other baking sheet then drizzle olive oil on top. Place both baking sheets in the oven to roast the vegetables.

After 10 minutes, remove the baking sheet with the peppers from the oven. Place the peppers in a zip lock bag and leave the vegetables to sweat for 10 minutes. Take out the peppers and slowly peel off the skin. Slice the peppers into strips and set aside.

After 30 minutes, take out the roasted cauliflower florets from the oven and set aside.

Heat the butter in a large saucepan over medium-high flame. Once the butter starts to heat up, add in the green onions, thyme, red pepper flakes, garlic powder, paprika, salt and pepper. Mix well.

Once the spices are cooked, pour in the coconut cream and chicken broth. Stir and let the mixture simmer. Add in the cauliflower and peppers and simmer for 10 minutes before turning off the heat.

Pour the chowder into a blender and pulse a few times. If you want the chowder to come out smoother, blend the mixture for 15 seconds. Pour into bowls and serve immediately.

This recipe yields 5 servings.

13. Low-Carb Zucchini Carbonara

Ingredients:
 3 medium zucchinis, peeled

1 cup chopped bacon

3 tablespoons freshly-chopped basil leaves

½cup grated parmesan cheese

1 egg

2 egg yolks, beaten

2 tablespoons heavy cream

Pinch of salt and ground black pepper Directions:

Place the zucchinis through a spiralizer to form long, spaghetti-like noodles. Transfer the noodles to a bowl and set aside.

Fry the chopped bacon in a pan over medium-high flame until golden brown. Remove the bacon but save the bacon fat for later.

Whisk together the egg and egg yolks and season it with salt and pepper. Blend in the parmesan cheese and heavy cream then set aside.

Place the zucchini noodles in the pan of bacon fat and cook over medium-high flame for 5 minutes. Add the egg mixture then cook for 2-3 minutes with constant stirring. Turn off the heat and transfer the pasta to a serving plate.

Top the dish with bacon bits and serve immediately.

This recipe yields 3 servings.

14. Pan-Fried Salmon with Zesty Balsamic Sauce

Ingredients:

2 150-gram salmon fillets

2 tablespoons white wine

1 tablespoon organic ketchup

1 tablespoon fish sauce

2 teaspoons olive oil

2 tablespoons coconut aminos

1 tablespoon balsamic vinegar

2 teaspoons chopped garlic

1 teaspoon chopped ginger

2 teaspoons organic honey

Directions:

Mix together coconut aminos, honey, fish sauce, balsamic vinegar, garlic and ginger in a bowl. Place the salmon fillets in the balsamic mixture and marinate for 15 minutes.

After 15 minutes, drain the liquid from the salmon fillets and set aside.

Heat the olive oil in a pan over medium-high flame. Once the oil is hot, place the salmon fillets on the pan, skin side down. Fry for 3 minutes, then slowly flip the fillets and cook for another 3 minutes. Pour the balsamic marinade into the pan and let it boil with the fish.

Take out the fried fish from the pan and set aside. Pour the ketchup and white wine into the boiling marinade and cook for 5 minutes or until the sauce has reduced. Turn off the heat and cool for 5 minutes.

Place the salmon fillets on a plate and drizzle the sauce over it. Serve immediately.

This recipe yields 2 servings.

Chapter 5:
Dinner Recipes

D inners are important in a ketogenic lifestyle: healthy dishes that are high in healthy fats will help keep you full throughout the night, thus preventing you from giving into cravings for high-carb midnight snacks.

1. Quick and Easy Grilled Chicken Teriyaki

Ingredients:

2 chicken breasts, skin removed

1 tablespoon olive oil

½ cup water

2 tablespoons organic honey

1 cup coconut aminos

1 teaspoon freshly-grated ginger

1 teaspoon garlic powder

Pinch of salt

Directions:

Pat the chicken breasts dry with a kitchen towel. Drizzle olive oil all over the chicken then place them on a grill pan. Cook each side of the chicken for 8-10 minutes over medium-high flame then set aside.

Whisk together water, honey, coconut aminos, ginger, garlic powder and salt in a saucepan and place the teriyaki mixture over medium flame. Boil the sauce for 7-10 minutes while constantly stirring it. Turn off the flame once the sauce has reduced.

Transfer the chicken breasts into the saucepan. Make sure to coat all side of the chicken with the teriyaki sauce. Arrange the chicken on a serving plate and serve with your favorite greens.

This recipe yields 2 servings.

2. Slow-Braised Oxtail Stew

Ingredients:

900 grams oxtail, sliced

2 cups homemade chicken broth

3 tablespoons tomato paste

3 garlic cloves, crushed

2 tablespoons coconut aminos

½ cup butter

1 teaspoon onion powder

1 teaspoon turmeric powder

Pinch of salt and ground black pepper

Directions:

Arrange the sliced oxtail in a crock pot and season it with onion powder, turmeric powder, salt, pepper and crushed garlic. Pour in the chicken broth, coconut aminos and tomato paste.

Cover the crock pot and set the temperature to low. Cook the meat for 7 hours.

Place the cooked oxtails on a serving bowl. Use an immersion blender to puree the braising liquid inside the
 pot. Pour the sauce over the oxtail slices and serve while hot.

This recipe makes 4 servings.

3. **Wheat-Free Pork and Veggie Sandwich**

Ingredients:

900 grams lean ground pork

½ cup tomato sauce

1 large white onion, minced

2 eggs

Slices of tomato and cucumber

1½ tablespoons melted butter

½teaspoon paprika

½ teaspoon chili powder Pinch of salt and black pepper Directions:

Place the chopped onions in a pan over medium-high heat then pour in the melted butter. Cook the onions for 3 minutes then let it cool.

In a large bowl, mix together the pork, tomato sauce, eggs and cooked onions. Season it with salt, pepper, chili powder and paprika then mix thoroughly. Divide the pork mixture into 6 patties and place them on a parchment-lined baking sheet. Bake the patties in a 350 ° F oven for 45 minutes.

Once the patties are cooked, remove it from the oven and allow them to cool. Slice each patty horizontally in the middle to make 2 loaves. Place a patty slice on a plate, top with cucumbers and tomatoes then cover it with the other patty. Serve immediately.

This recipe yields 6 servings.

4. <u>Grilled Tilapia Fillet with Arugula Salad</u>

Ingredients:

3 Tilapia fillets

2 tablespoons lime zest

1 teaspoon sea salt

1 tablespoon lemon pepper seasoning

1 teaspoon garlic powder

1 tablespoon melted coconut oil

2 cups arugula, washed and drained

1 tablespoon lemon juice

1 tablespoon olive oil

1 teaspoon honey

Directions:

To make the arugula salad, mix together the arugula leaves, lemon juice, olive oil and honey until the leaves are well-coated. Set this aside.

In another bowl, combine the lime zest, sea salt, lemon pepper seasoning and garlic powder. Place the tilapia fillets into the spice mixture and coat evenly.

Grease the grill pan with the coconut oil and place it over medium-high flame. Place the tilapia on the grill pan and cook each side for 3-5 minutes.

Once the fillets are cooked, arrange them on a serving plate. Serve the tilapia with the prepared arugula salad.

This recipe yields 3 servings.

5. <u>Slow Cooker Roast Beef with Honey Citrus Sauce</u>

Ingredients:

900 grams beef chuck roast

2 tablespoons fresh lime juice

2 tablespoons fresh orange juice

1 tablespoon honey

½ cup olive oil

3 garlic cloves, minced

½cup chopped cilantro

1 large shallot, minced

1 teaspoon chili powder

2 teaspoons oregano powder

2 teaspoons sea salt ¼ teaspoon cumin ¼ teaspoon coriander ¼ cup water Directions:

Place the beef chuck inside the slow cooker. Let it stand for 20-30 minutes.

In a food processor, mix together the lime juice, orange juice, honey, olive oil, cilantro, shallot, chili powder, oregano, salt, cumin and coriander. Pour the mixture into the pot, making sure to coat the beef evenly. Pour in the water then cover the pot.

Set the temperature to high and cook the beef for 4 hours, turning the meat every hour. After 4 hours, turn off the slow cooker and tilt the cover of the pot to let the heat dissipate. Leave it for 20 minutes.

Remove the beef from the pot and place it on a serving plate. Slice the meat according to preferred thickness and pour the citrus sauce over it. Serve immediately.

This recipe yields 4-5 servings.

6. Coconut Fish Fingers with Garlic Mayo Dip

Ingredients:

450 grams cream dory, sliced into strips

¾cup shredded coconut

2 medium eggs, beaten

4 tablespoons olive oil

 Pinch of salt and black pepper For the Dip:

1 teaspoon garlic powder
3 tablespoons mayonnaise

½ teaspoon honey Directions:

Wash the fish strips and drain completely. Place the eggs in a bowl and put the shredded coconut on a separate plate.

Heat the olive oil in a pan over medium high flame.

Dip the fish finger into the egg mixture then roll it on the grated coconut. Repeat this procedure again to ensure that the fish is evenly coated.

Place the fish finger into the pan and cook until the sides have turned golden brown. Lay the fish finger on a wire rack to cool. Arrange the fish fingers on a serving plate and serve immediately.

For the dip, mix together the mayonnaise, garlic powder and honey. Pour the mixture in a sauce bowl and serve.

This recipe yields 4 servings.

7. <u>Turkey and Vegetable Pot Pie</u>

Ingredients:

1 cup leftover turkey meat, diced

1 egg, beaten

1 cup diced celery

1 cup diced zucchini

1 cup homemade chicken broth

Pinch of salt and ground black pepper

For the Crust:

2 large eggs

½ cup coconut oil 1½ cups almond flour

½ cup coconut flour Pinch of sea salt Directions:

To make the crust, combine the almond and coconut flours in a bowl then season it with salt. Add in coconut oil and egg. Knead through the mixture until a soft dough forms.

Separate the dough mixture into 2 balls. Place each dough ball in between 2 sheets of wax paper then use a rolling pin to flatten them. Place one flattened dough in a lightly-greased pie pan and spread the dough until the sides of the pan are covered. Bake this in a 325 ° F oven for 6-8 minutes.

While the pie crust is baking, place the turkey, egg, celery, zucchini and chicken broth in a saucepan and simmer over medium flame for 8 minutes. Season it with salt and pepper. Once the liquids have reduced, turn off the heat and set aside.

Once the pie crust is ready, remove it from the oven and let it cool for 3-5 minutes. Pour the turkey mixture into the pie crust. Slowly put the remaining flattened dough on top of the pie. Make sure to seal the sides of the pie but do make small vents on top by poking it with a fork or knife.

Place the pie in the oven and bake for 45-50 minutes. Slice into equal portions and serve.

This recipe yields 8 servings.

8. Carb-Friendly Chili Bowl
Ingredients:

900 grams ground beef

7 cups spinach leaves

1 green bell pepper, deseeded and chopped

1 red bell pepper, deseeded and chopped

1 medium onion, chopped

1 cup tomato sauce

1 tablespoon chili powder

1 tablespoon cumin

2 teaspoons cayenne pepper

1 teaspoon garlic powder

½teaspoon curry powder

1 tablespoon olive oil

2 tablespoons cottage cheese

Pinch of salt and ground black pepper Directions:

Place the ground beef in a pot and start cooking it over high flame. Stir every few minutes to prevent it from burning.

While the beef starts to cook, heat the olive oil in a large pan over medium flame. Add in the onions and bell peppers and sauté for 10 minutes. Add in the spinach leaves and cook for 10 more minutes. Season with salt and pepper and set aside.

Season the beef with chili powder, cumin, cayenne pepper, garlic powder and curry powder. Lower the flame to medium and continue cooking for 20-25 minutes.

Once the beef is cooked, add the cooked vegetables and tomato sauce into the pot and mix well. Simmer for 10 minutes then turn off the heat. Sprinkle some cottage cheese on top and serve while hot.

This recipe yields 8 servings.

9. Barbecued Short Ribs with Asian Spices

Ingredients:

6 short rib flanks

2 tablespoons fish sauce

2 tablespoons coconut aminos

1 tablespoon oyster sauce

2 tablespoons rice vinegar

½teaspoon red pepper flakes

1 teaspoon minced ginger

1 teaspoon minced garlic

½teaspoon sesame seeds

½teaspoon onion powder

1 tablespoon salt

Directions:

Combine the rice vinegar, oyster sauce, fish sauce, and coconut aminos in a large bowl. Place the short ribs in the marinade and let it sit for 1 hour.

In a separate bowl, mix the pepper flakes, ginger, garlic, onion powder, salt, and sesame seeds. Rub the spice mix into the marinated short ribs.

Place the short ribs on the barbecue grill and cook each side for 5 minutes. Remove the meat from the grill and slice into smaller portions. Serve while hot.

This recipe yields 6 servings.

10. Low-Carb Vegetarian Pan Pizza

Ingredients:

2 tablespoons psyllium husk powder

4 eggs

1 teaspoon Italian seasoning

3 tablespoons parmesan cheese

3 teaspoons olive oil

Pinch of salt

2 tablespoons freshly-chopped basil leaves

1 cup cheddar cheese, grated

4 tablespoons tomato sauce

Directions:

For the pizza crust batter, combine eggs, psyllium husk, parmesan cheese and salt in a blender and mix well.

Set aside.

Heat the olive oil in a large pan over medium-high flame. Pour half of the pizza crust batter into the pan and let it cook for 2-3 minutes. Flip the pizza crust and cook the remaining side for 2 minutes. Make another pizza crust using the same procedure.

Place both pizza crusts on a baking sheet. Spoon equal portions of tomato sauce, grated cheese and chopped basil on the pizza crust. Bake the pizza in a 225 ° F oven for 5-10 minutes.

This recipe yields 2 servings.

11.   Oven-Baked Rib-eye Steak

Ingredients:

3 medium rib-eye steaks

3 tablespoons butter

1 tablespoon paprika

1 tablespoon garlic powder

Pinch of salt and ground black pepper

Directions:

Rub the rib-eye steaks with salt, pepper, paprika and garlic powder. Place it in a lightly-greased baking dish.

Bake the steaks in a 250 ° F oven for 45 minutes.

Use a cooking thermometer to check for the steak's doneness. If it reaches 120 ° F then the steak is ready.

Remove the steak from the oven and let it stand for 5 minutes.

Heat the butter in a pan over medium flame. Once the oil is hot, place the steaks on the pan and sear each side of the meat for 30-40 seconds. Serve immediately.
 This recipe yields 3 servings.

12.   Pan-Fried Chicken Breast with Citrus Sauce

Ingredients:

3 chicken breast halves, skin intact

2 cups kale leaves, washed and stems discarded

½ teaspoon butter

2 tablespoons heavy cream

3 tablespoons olive oil

2 tablespoons organic honey

½teaspoon dried rosemary

1 cup fresh orange juice

Pinch of salt and ground black pepper Directions:

Season the chicken breast with salt and pepper. Place it in a pan over medium-high flame and cook each side for 8-10 minutes. Set aside.

While the chicken breasts are cooking, heat the olive oil in a pan over medium flame. Add in the rosemary, orange juice and honey and simmer for 5-7 minutes. Pour in the heavy cream and cook for 3 minutes. Turn off the heat and set aside.

Place the butter and kale leaves on the same pan where the chicken breast was cooked. Cook the greens for 3-5 minutes or until the leaves wilt.

Transfer the wilted greens on a plate and arrange the chicken breasts on top of it. Pour the orange sauce on top of the dish. Serve immediately.

This recipe yields 3 servings.

13.   Flaky Coconut Crusted Shrimp with Tangy Chili Dip

Ingredients:

450 grams shrimps, peeled and deveined

2 tablespoons coconut flour

1 cup dried coconut flakes

2 egg whites

1 red chili, minced

½cup crushed pineapple

1 tablespoon lemon juice

1½ tablespoons white vinegar Pinch of red pepper flakes Directions:

Preheat the oven to 225 ° F and line a baking sheet with parchment paper.

Beat the egg whites until soft white peaks form. Set this aside. Place the coconut flour and coconut flakes in separate bowls.

Dip each shrimp in this order: coconut flour, egg whites then coconut flakes. Arrange the shrimps on the baking sheet until all seafood has been coated. Place the shrimps in the oven and bake for 5 minutes. Turn off the oven

 and arrange the shrimp on a serving platter.

To make the dip, mix together the crushed pineapple, lemon juice, vinegar and pepper flakes. Place the mixture in a sauce bowl and serve alongside the coconut shrimp.

This recipe yields 4 servings.

14.   Crock Pot Leg of Lamb with Fresh Herb Sauce

Ingredients:

900 grams lamb leg

2 tablespoons Dijon mustard

3 garlic cloves, minced

4 fresh thyme sprigs

¼ cup olive oil

1 teaspoon fresh rosemary

1 tablespoon organic honey

6 mint leaves

Pinch of salt and ground black pepper

Directions:

Make 3-4 hollow slices into the lamb leg and place equal amounts of garlic and rosemary into the slits. Place the lamb in the slow cooker and season it with salt, pepper, honey and mustard.

Cover the crock pot and cook the leg on low for 7 hours. After 7 hours, add in the mint leaves and thyme then cook the meat for 1 hour.

Remove the lamb from the pot and slice. Serve hot.

This recipe yields 6 servings.

Chapter 6:
Snack Recipes

S nacking is definitely allowed in the ketogenic diet. Just remember to use organic ingredients such as vegetables, meats and high-fat oils to create healthier versions of your favorite chips, crackers or spreads.

1. Spicy Baked Zucchini Chips

Ingredients:

1 large zucchini, sliced thinly

1 teaspoon paprika

½ teaspoon chili powder

3 teaspoons coconut oil

½ teaspoon ground white pepper

½ teaspoon salt

Directions:

Place the zucchini slices in a colander, sprinkle salt over it and let it stand in the sink for 1 hour. This allows water from the zucchini to drain out completely. Once the water has been completely drained, pat the zucchini slices with a paper towel and set aside.

Line a baking sheet with parchment paper and preheat the oven to 300 ° F. Grease the parchment with a little oil. Arrange the zucchini slices evenly on the baking sheet. Brush some oil on the vegetable slices then sprinkle it salt, pepper, paprika and chili powder.

Place the zucchini in the oven and bake for 30 minutes. Turn off the oven but let the vegetable chips continue cooking for 45 minutes.

This recipe yields 3-4 servings.

2. Garlicky Pork Chips

Ingredients:

200 grams freshly-sliced prosciutto, cut into thin strips

1 teaspoon garlic powder

Directions:

Preheat the oven to 350 ° F and prepare a parchment-lined baking sheet.

Place the prosciutto on the baking sheet. Sprinkle garlic powder on top of the prosciutto. Place the sheet inside the oven and bake for 10-15 minutes. Make sure to keep an eye on the prosciutto to prevent it from burning.

Once the prosciutto is golden brown, remove it from the oven and let it cool on a wire rack. Lightly tap or tear the prosciutto to make chips. Serve immediately.

This recipe yields 3 servings.

3. Extra Spicy Devilled Eggs

Ingredients:

8 hard-boiled eggs, peeled

1 tablespoon Dijon mustard

4 tablespoons mayonnaise

1 teaspoon hot sauce
Pinch of paprika

Directions:

Slice each hard-boiled egg in half and scoop out the yolk. Place the yolks in a bowl and set aside the whites.

Add mustard, mayonnaise, hot sauce and paprika to the yolks and mash the ingredients together. Place the yolk mixture in a piping bag. Place 8 egg white halves on a plate. Pipe the yolk mixture beginning from the hollow portion of the egg white moving upwards. Place the other egg white halves on top of the devilled eggs. Serve warm.

This recipe yields 8 servings.

4. Nutty Spiced Kale Chips

Ingredients:

2 bunches of kale, washed and stems removed

1 tablespoon honey

2 tablespoons olive oil

½cup lemon juice

½cup almond butter

½cup peanut butter

½tablespoon coconut aminos

½cup apple cider vinegar

1 tablespoon balsamic vinegar

1 red bell pepper, deseeded and chopped

¼ cup nutritional yeast

1 teaspoon garlic powder Pinch of salt and black pepper Directions:

Chop the kale into bite-sized pieces and place them on a

layer of paper towels to dry. Set this aside. Preheat the

oven to 200 ° F and line a baking sheet with parchment

paper. Set this aside.

While the kale leaves are drying, place all of the spices, oils, nut butters and vinegars into a food processor. Add in the honey, yeast, bell pepper, lemon juice and coconut aminos. Blend the ingredients until a creamy paste is produced. Season the mixture with salt and pepper.

Pour the nut butter mixture in a large mixing bowl. Add in the kale leaves and toss until the leaves are evenly coated. Arrange the kale leaves on the baking sheet, making sure to not overcrowd it. Place it in the oven and bake the kale for 3 hours or until the leaves are crispy.

This recipe yields 4 servings.

5. <u>Hot and Spicy Turnip Fries</u>

Ingredients:

2 turnips, peeled and sliced into thick strips

½ teaspoon chili powder

½ teaspoon paprika

1 tablespoon olive oil

Pinch of salt and black pepper
Directions:

Preheat the oven to 375 ° F and prepare a parchment-lined baking sheet.

Place the turnip fries in a large bowl and drizzle olive oil on top. Season the vegetable with chili powder, paprika, salt and pepper then toss for an even coating.

Arrange the turnip fries evenly on the baking sheet and place it in the oven. Bake for 25-30 minutes or until the turnip fries become light brown in color. You may also check for the tenderness of the fries by poking them with a skewer.

This recipe yields 4 servings.

6. Cheesy Baked Sugar Snap Peas

Ingredients:

4 cups sugar snap peas, washed and drained

2 tablespoons grated parmesan cheese

2 teaspoons olive oil

½ teaspoon garlic powder Pinch of sea salt

Mayonnaise and lemon juice for dipping Directions:

Arrange the snap peas on a baking sheet and drizzle olive oil on top of it. Season the vegetables with salt and garlic powder then sprinkle the grated cheese on top.

Place the snap peas in a 425 ° F oven and bake for 15 minutes. After 15 minutes, flip the snap peas over and continue baking for another 15 minutes.

Arrange the baked snap peas on a plate. Make a mayo and lemon juice dip to complement the flavors of the vegetables. Serve hot.

This recipe yields 2-3 servings.

7. Bacon and Sausage Knots

Ingredients:

10 Italian Sausages, sliced into 4

20 bacon strips, halved

2 cups olive oil

20 toothpicks Directions:

Heat the olive oil in a pan over high flame.

Wrap each sausage piece with bacon, covering the sides and the sliced areas. Place toothpicks to secure the bacon around the sausage.

Deep fry the sausages for 4 minutes or until the bacon turns golden brown. Lay the snacks on paper towels to drain any excess oil.

This recipe yields 10 servings.

8. Crispy Brussels Sprouts with Hot Mayo Sauce

Ingredients:

4 cups Brussels sprouts, washed and drained
 2 teaspoons lemon juice

¾ cup mayonnaise

2 teaspoons hot sauce

3 cups olive oil

Directions:

Slice the Brussels sprouts in quarters and set aside.

Heat the olive oil in a deep frying pan over high flame. Deep fry the vegetables in 6-8 batches. Place the fried vegetables on a layer of paper towels to drain excess oil.

To make the sauce, combine the lemon juice, mayonnaise, hot sauce and salt in a bowl. Whisk until a smooth texture forms.

Arrange the fried Brussels sprouts on a large plate. Drizzle the mayonnaise over the vegetables and lightly toss.

Serve while hot.

This recipe makes 12 servings.

9. Creamy Ham and Asparagus Rollups

Ingredients:

6 large slices of cooked ham

6 asparagus sticks, bottoms trimmed off

3 cups cottage cheese

18 toothpicks Directions:

Boil the asparagus sticks in water for 5 minutes. Once the vegetables are tender, remove them from the heat and drain the water completely.

Lay a slice of ham on the chopping board. Spoon a half cup of cottage cheese on the ham, then place an asparagus stick at the bottom part. Slowly roll the ham upwards. Slice the dish into 3 and secure each portion with a toothpick. Serve immediately.

This recipe yields 6 servings.

10. Celery Sticks with Homemade Nut Butter Dip

Ingredients:

2 cups celery sticks

1 cup almonds, toasted

2 cups macadamia nuts, toasted

1 teaspoon organic honey

¼ teaspoon sea salt ½ teaspoon vanilla Directions:

Place the almonds, macadamia nuts, honey, salt and vanilla in a food processor. Blend the ingredients for 3 minutes. Pour the nut butter in a jar or sauce bowl.

Arrange the celery sticks on a plate. Serve with a side of homemade nut butter.

This recipe yields 3-4 servings.

11. Light and Healthy Spinach Crackers

Ingredients:

150 grams frozen spinach, thawed and drained

¼ cup coconut flour

½ cup grated parmesan cheese 1½ cups almond flour

½cup flaxseed meal

½teaspoon red pepper flakes

½teaspoon cumin powder

¼ cup softened butter ½ teaspoon sea salt Directions:

Boil the spinach leaves and a cup of water in a saucepan for 1 minute. Drain the spinach leaves and use your hand to squeeze out any excess liquid from the leaves. Place the spinach in a food processor and blend for 30 seconds. Set aside.

Combine the coconut flour, almond flour, parmesan cheese and softened butter in a bowl. Mix well. Season the dry ingredients with salt, cumin and red pepper flakes.

Add in the ground spinach and mix until a soft dough forms. Place the dough in between two sheets of wax paper and use a rolling pin to flatten it. Transfer the flattened dough on a parchment-lined baking sheet and continue rolling it to the sides of the sheet.

Slice the dough into squares and place it in the oven. Bake it for 30 minutes at 250 ° F.

This recipe yields 8 servings.

12. Yummy Bacon and Egg Bites

Ingredients:

2 medium hard-boiled egg, peeled

1 tablespoon mayonnaise

2 tablespoons softened butter

2 bacon slices, cooked

Pinch of salt and ground black pepper

Directions:

Chop the cooked bacon into small pieces and set aside.

Combine the hard-boiled eggs, butter and mayonnaise in a bowl. Mash the ingredients together and season it with salt and pepper. Form the mixture into 3 balls and roll it into the chopped bacon. Serve immediately.

This recipe yields 3 servings.

13.   **Baked Coconut Crisps**

Ingredients:

4 cups unsweetened coconut flakes

1 teaspoon cinnamon

2 tablespoons Erythritol

1 teaspoon vanilla extract
4 tablespoons coconut oil, melted

Pinch of sea salt

Directions:

Preheat the oven to 350 ° F and prepare a parchment-lined baking sheet.

Place the coconut flakes in a large bowl. Add in the cinnamon, Erythritol, vanilla, coconut oil and salt. Toss the ingredients together.

Transfer the coconut flakes on the baking sheet and place it in the oven. Bake for 5 minutes or until the flakes turn light brown. Remove the coconut from the oven and let it cool on a wire rack.

This recipe yields 8 servings.

14.   **Low-Carb Caprese Salad Sticks**

Ingredients:

4 cups small mozzarella balls

1 cup mixed olives, pitted

4 cups cherry tomatoes

4 tablespoons fresh basil leaves

4 tablespoons pesto sauce

1 teaspoon olive oil

4 skewers Directions:

In a small bowl, combine the mozzarella and pesto. Mix well until the mozzarella is evenly coated.

Get a skewer and pierce a tomato through it, followed by a mozzarella ball, an olive and a basil leaf. Do another row of the same ingredients. Create 3 more Caprese salad sticks then arrange them on a plate. Drizzle olive oil on top and serve.

This recipe yields 4 servings.

Chapter 7:
Dessert Recipes

Combining small amounts of fruit, chocolate, natural sweeteners, oils and organic flours helps create nutritious and delectable ketogenic-friendly desserts. But do remember that small amounts of dessert yield better results, especially around the waistline.

1. Freezer–Friendly Chocolate Pudding

Ingredients:

4 tablespoons cocoa powder

2 cups full fat coconut milk

1 ½ teaspoon stevia powder extract

3 tablespoons water

2 tablespoons powdered gelatin

Directions:

Place the cocoa powder, stevia and coconut milk in a saucepan over medium heat. Slowly mix until the cocoa is dissolved.

In a separate bowl, blend the gelatin and water until the gelatin dissolves. Pour the gelatin mixture into the cocoa mixture and mix thoroughly.

Once the pudding mixture starts to heat up, turn off the stove. Pour the pudding mixture into 4 ramekins or pudding cups and place them in the freezer to set.

This recipe yields 4 servings.

2. Luscious Coconut Brownies

Ingredients:

1 cup cocoa powder

2 teaspoons stevia powder extract

2 large eggs

1 cup almond flour

½cup shredded coconut

1 teaspoon vanilla

½teaspoon baking soda

½cup chopped almonds

½cup coconut milk

1 cup coconut oil, melted

Directions:

Prepare a square baking pan by brushing it lightly with olive oil.
Preheat the oven to 350 ° F.

Place the baking soda, coconut and almond flour in a mixing bowl and blend thoroughly. In another bowl, whisk together eggs, vanilla, stevia, cocoa powder, coconut milk and coconut oil. Combine both mixtures together then gradually fold in the almonds.

Pour the brownie mixture into the pan and bake in the oven for 30 minutes. Let the brownies cool before slicing it into 9 squares.
This recipe yields 9 servings.

3. **Chocolate Almond Squares**

Ingredients:

120 grams dark chocolate chips

1 cup shredded coconut

1 cup almond flour

3 tablespoons coconut oil

1 ½ cups almond butter

¾ cup coconut sugar Directions:

Heat the almond butter and 2 tablespoons of the coconut oil in a saucepan over medium-low flame. Once the ingredients have melted, turn off the heat. Fold in the almond flour, coconut sugar and shredded coconut into the saucepan and mix well.

Pour the almond mixture into a square-sized baking pan and set aside.

Heat the chocolate chips and remaining coconut oil in a saucepan over medium flame until the chocolate melts.
Mix well.

Pour the melted chocolate mixture on top of the almond mixture, making sure that the top of the dessert is evenly-coated. Refrigerate for 2 hours then slice the dessert into 20 almond squares.

This recipe yields 10 servings.

4. Chewy Chocolate Zucchini Brownies

Ingredients:

1 cup gluten free semi-sweet chocolate chips

1 ½ cups shredded zucchini, drained

1 cup almond butter

1 large egg

1 teaspoon cinnamon

1 teaspoon baking soda

½ cup organic honey Directions:

Preheat the oven to 350 ° F and lightly grease a 9x9 baking pan.

Combine the zucchini, chocolate chips, egg, almond butter, honey, baking soda and cinnamon in a mixing bowl. Pour the mixture into the baking pan.

Bake the brownies for 45 minutes. Slice into squares and serve.

This recipe yields 9 servings.

5. Coconut Pudding with Fresh Berries

Ingredients:

2 cups full-fat coconut milk

1 cup fresh strawberries, stems removed

½ cup blueberries
½ tablespoon stevia

½teaspoon vanilla

3 tablespoons flaxseeds

Directions:

Place the coconut milk, strawberries, mangoes, stevia, vanilla and flaxseeds in a blender and pulse until the ingredients are mixed well.

Pour the mixture into 2 bowls and place it in the freezer for 1 hour. Serve chilled.

This recipe yields 2 servings.

6. Almond Coconut Fat Bombs

Ingredients:

2 tablespoons almond butter

1 cup softened cold-pressed coconut oil

3 tablespoons unsweetened cocoa powder

2 tablespoons organic honey

1 teaspoon vanilla

½ teaspoon sea salt

1 cup shredded coconut

Directions:

Place the almond butter, coconut oil, cocoa powder, honey, vanilla and sea salt in a food processor and mix until smooth and creamy.

Form the mixture into 16 candy balls. Roll each ball into the shredded coconut and place on a parchment-lined sheet. Refrigerate the candies for 1 hour then transfer them in an airtight container.

This recipe yields 8 servings.

7. **Frozen Watermelon Creamsicles**

Ingredients:

2 cups watermelon chunks, deseeded

1 ¾ cups full-fat coconut milk

1 teaspoon vanilla

1 tablespoon organic honey

Directions:

Puree the watermelon in a food processor and pour it into a bowl, making sure to discard seeds. Place the fruit puree back into the food processor then pour in the honey, vanilla and coconut milk. Process until the mixture becomes smooth and creamy.

Pour the watermelon mixture into 4 molds and place popsicle sticks through the dessert. Place the popsicles in the freezer for 4-5 hours.

This recipe yields 4 servings.

8. **Low-Carb Cinnamon Pumpkin Blondie**

Ingredients:

1 teaspoon cinnamon
1 cup canned pumpkin puree

½cup organic honey

1 cup almond butter

1 teaspoon baking soda

1 tablespoon melted coconut oil

1 egg

1 teaspoon vanilla extract Directions:

Place the pumpkin puree in a mixing bowl. Add in the cinnamon, honey, almond butter, baking soda, coconut oil, egg and vanilla extract. Mix well.

Pour the batter into a square 8x8 baking pan. Bake the dish in a preheated 350 ° F oven for 30 minutes. Slice into squares and serve.

This recipe yields 9 servings.

9. Watermelon & Cucumber Sorbet

Ingredients:

1 ½ cup diced cucumber meat

4 cups watermelon chunks, deseeded

2 tablespoons lime juice

2 tablespoons Erythritol

1 cup crushed ice

Directions:

Combine the cucumber, watermelon, lime juice, Erythritol and ice in a blender and mix for 15-20 seconds. Pour the mixture into a stainless bowl and freeze for 2 hours.

Take out the sorbet from the freezer and let it stand for 5 minutes. Scoop the sorbet into individual cups and serve.

This recipe yields 3 servings.

10. Heavenly Chocolate Bacon Strips

Ingredients:

16 bacon slices (thin slices)

2 tablespoons Erythritol

1 tablespoon coconut oil

1 teaspoon maple syrup

1 cup dark chocolate chips

Pinch of cinnamon powder

Directions:

Preheat the oven to 275 ° F and line a baking sheet with parchment paper.

In a small bowl combine the cinnamon powder and Erythritol. Sprinkle the mixture on both sides of the bacon.

Arrange the bacon on the baking sheet and bake it in the oven for 60 minutes. The bacon should be crisp and golden brown in color. To make the chocolate coating, melt the chocolate chips with the coconut oil and maple syrup using a double boiler. Stir until the chocolate melts and is warm to the touch.

Take out the bacon from the oven and let it cool for 5 minutes. Use a spoon to coat the bacon with the melted chocolate. Let the chocolate-covered bacon harden on a baking sheet. Place the bacon strips in the fridge.

This recipe yields 8 servings.

11.   Vanilla Meringue Bites

Ingredients:

½teaspoon vanilla extract

½teaspoon apple cider vinegar

1 ½ tablespoon Erythritol

4 egg whites Directions:

Preheat the oven to 275 ° F and prepare a parchment-lined cookie sheet.

Whisk the egg whites using an electric mixer and place it on medium-low speed for 2 minutes. Once the eggs become foamy, gradually mix in the apple cider vinegar, vanilla and Erythritol. Beat the whites until glossy white peaks form.

Place the meringue mixture in a piping bag and pipe 24 small mounds on the cookie sheet. Bake the meringue in the oven for 15 minutes then lower the temperature to 200 ° F. Continue baking the dessert for 1 hour. Let it cool in room temperature before serving.

This recipe yields 6 servings.

12.   High Fiber Blueberry Milkshake

Ingredients:

1 cup fresh blueberries

1 cup coconut milk

½ cup almond milk

2 tablespoons melted coconut oil

1 ½ tablespoons chia seeds

2 drops liquid stevia

1 teaspoon vanilla extract

½ cup crushed ice Directions:

Pour the coconut milk, almond milk, vanilla and coconut oil into a blender and pulse. Add in the blueberries, chia seeds, stevia and ice and process until smooth. Pour the milkshake into individual glasses and serve.

This recipe yields 2 servings.

13.   Chocolate Peppermint Bark

Ingredients:

4 tablespoons coconut oil, melted

½ teaspoon peppermint extract

2 tablespoons unsweetened cocoa powder
 2 tablespoons Erythritol

2 tablespoons heavy cream

2 tablespoons toasted almonds, chopped

Pinch of sea salt

Directions:

Combine coconut oil, peppermint extract, cocoa powder, Erythritol, salt and toasted almonds in a bowl. Fold in the heavy cream and mix until the texture becomes silky.

Pour the chocolate mixture in a lined baking pan then place it in the freezer for 2-3 hours.

Break apart the chocolate bark into bite-sized pieces. Serve frozen.

This recipe yields 4 servings.

14.   Mini Strawberry Cheesecake Balls

Ingredients:

¾ cups softened cream cheese

½ cup frozen strawberries, thawed

1 tablespoon almond extract ¼ cup butter

2 tablespoons Erythritol

1 cup almond flour Directions:

Let the butter and cream cheese melt in a bowl at room temperature for 45 minutes. Once melted, place the ingredients in a food processor.

Add in the almond extract, Erythritol and strawberries. Mix the ingredients until the mixture turns creamy.

Use a spoon to make small round balls from the cheesecake mixture. Roll it on a plate with almond flour then place it in a small cupcake liner.

Freeze the dessert for 2 hours. Serve chilled.

This recipe yields 10-12 servings.

Conclusion

Thank you again for downloading this book!

I hope this book was able to encourage you to adopt an effective ketogenic meal planning system based on the low-carbohydrate recipes that were shown in the preceding chapters

Moreover, I hope that you will regularly practice a ketogenic lifestyle as this will not only help you achieve a healthy weight, but will also create a positively life-changing balance between the mind, body, and soul.

The next step is to try out more ketogenic recipes from this book and create a meal plan that will best suit your lifestyle and health goals.

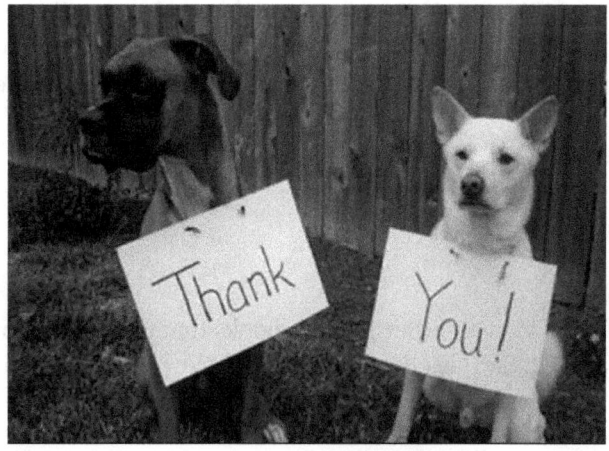

Finally, if you enjoyed this book, then I'd like to ask you for a favor, would you be kind enough to leave a review for this book on Amazon? It'd be greatly appreciated!

Click here to leave a review for this book on Amazon!

or go to http://amzn.to/1YwE9N1

Thank you and good luck!

Preview Of 'Running Guide for Beginners: How to Start Running for Weight Loss and Increase Endurance'

Chapter 1 – Benefits of Running

For most people, running does not seem to be an effective way to lose weight. Although going to the gym and lifting heavy dumbbells can really help in toning your muscles, it doesn't mean that jogging a few laps around the park is useless.

In fact, running will not just strengthen your leg muscles; it will also improve your bone density, relieve stress, and even fortify your immune system. Can you believe that a *simple physical exercise* can do so much? If not, check out these other compelling reasons why should start running today!

1. Keeps depression at bay

When you are depressed, it is understandable that you will feel too lazy or weak to run outdoors. However, it is highly recommended that you try running because it'll definitely remove the blues out of your system.

Click here to check out the rest of "Running Guide for Begineers" on Amazon.

Or go to: amzn.to/20HlVsr
Check Out Other Books

Below you'll find some of other popular books that are popular on Amazon and Kindle as well. Simply click on the links below to check them out.

Running Guide for Beginners: How to Start Running for Weight Loss and Increase Endurance
- Chris Douglas

STRETCHING: Pre and Post Running Stretching Exercises
- Chris Douglas

Meditation and Mindfulness for Beginners: Easy, Simple and Practical Steps to Relieve Stress, Anxiety and Achieve Peace and Happiness
- Chris Douglas

CPSIA information can be obtained
at www.ICGtesting.com
Printed in the USA
BVHW041515110321
602278BV00012B/1295

9 781914 418303